The Intersection of Cr
A Study on Yoga's Effect

Tracy R. Shell

TABLE OF CONTENTS

Page

LIST OF TABLES AND FIGURES

Tables

Figures

ABSTRACT

Creativity is perhaps the most important factor contributing to human happiness and adaptation, and yet there is little known about initiating and maintaining creative states commonly referred to as flow. In a time of global population expansion, economic uncertainty and political chaos, the challenges we currently face are without precedent. Creativity is implicated in workplace success, healthy psychological functioning, and the maintenance of healthy interpersonal relationships (Csikszentmihalyi, 1990). Psychologists, medical doctors and researchers are beginning to recognize the healing power of creative flow and understand its ability to advance the field of psychology and improve people's lives. This research is an investigation into the mind-body connection through a practice of Hatha Yoga and its impact on the creative process. This study purposes to evaluate the efficacy of integrating a practice of Hatha Yoga with positive psychology, mindfulness, and art therapy directives into an intervention to beneficially influence the creative process and increase overall well-being in adults.

Chapter I

Introduction

In 1950 J.P. Guilford gave a Presidential address to the American Psychological Association (APA), challenging them to pay attention to what he called a neglected but extremely important attribute, creativity (Plunker, 2001). In his speech Guilford reported "Less than .02% of the entries in *Psychological Abstracts* up to 1950 focused on creativity" (Sternberg & Lubart, 1999, p. 3), stating that "The neglect of this subject by psychologists is appalling" (Guilford, 1950). Creativity is important to society but has traditionally been one of psychology's orphans. It is a topic that is marginally covered in introductory psychology textbooks, and major psychology departments rarely offer courses dedicated to the specific study of creativity. In terms of academic positions there are minimal listings for positions in the study of creativity and departments are not typically organized into a division for the study (unlike divisions studying cognitive, behavioral, social or clinical psychology). Few resources have been invested into the study of creativity, relative to its importance to the field of psychology and to the world. (Sternberg & Lubart, 1999).

The work of J.P. Guilford, E. Torrance and Calvin Taylor, among many others, helped to attract greater attention to creativity, but it was not until the initiation of positive psychology that creativity research began to flourish. Positive psychology takes root in humanistic approaches and is the study of how human beings prosper in the face of adversity (Froh, 2004). Its goals are to identify and enhance the human strengths and virtues that make life worth living, and allow individuals and communities to thrive (Seligman & Csikszentmihalyi, 2000). Mihaly Csikszentmihalyi was a young man in the aftermath of World War II and became one of positive psychology's leading proponents. While investigating the roots of happiness his studies led him to conclude that happiness was an internal state of being. It was this understanding that led him to *flow*.

Flow is a construct developed by Csíkszentmihályi that describes a psychological state of optimal attention and engagement (Chilton, 2013). His popular book, Flow: The Psychology of Optimal Experience (1990) is based on the premise that happiness levels can be shifted through the introduction of more flow. "Happiness" he says "is not a rigid state that can't be changed. On the contrary, happiness takes a committed effort to be manifested. After the baseline set point, there is a percentage of happiness that every individual has the responsibility to take control of" (Csikszentmihalyi, 1990, p. 104).

Problem Statement

Creativity is a topic of wide scope that is important at both the individual and societal levels. At an individual level creativity is relevant for solving problems and creating happiness and meaning in life. At a societal level creativity can bring about scientific and medical breakthroughs, new movements in art, technology innovation and improved governments and social programs (Sternberg & Lubart, 1999). Against a backdrop of uncertainty and unprecedented change, a new picture of success and survival is beginning to emerge in the modern era. At the center of this essential skillset for the future lies creative thinking, and yet there is still little known about how to harness and maintain creative states.

Purpose of the Study

This study seeks to provide a more in-depth understanding of creative flow, to strengthen the mind-body connection and to promote general well-being in adults. The study implements an intervention of Hatha Yoga while integrating the principal elements of positive psychology, mindfulness and art therapy directives. The yoga practice provides physiological and psychological benefits through the combination of conscious movement, breathing and meditation. Mindfulness is a core component of the yoga practice and provides participants with valuable life skills for strengthening the mind-body connection (Ross & Thomas, 2010). Positive psychology presents the framework for optimal psychological states by highlighting the key elements that contribute to flow consciousness. Art therapy directives were implemented as a method of understanding the effectiveness of the yoga intervention and to promote reflection, self-awareness and integration of the total experience.

Objectives

The goal of this research study was investigate the impact of a yoga practice on flow states, to strengthen the mind-body connection and to promote overall well-being in individuals. It was hypothesized that participants' creative capacities would be altered and that a reduction in stress would occur through a weekly practice of Hatha Yoga, coupled with the art experiential of mandala making.

Curriculum:

- Provide positive psychological experiences that promote happiness and well-being, emotionally and physically.
- Provide mind-body educational experiences that promote health benefits of practicing yoga and meditation.
- Explore component of the creative process.
- Provide an artistic outlet to promote self-reflection, self-awareness, and the integration of techniques learned in the curriculum.
- Decrease stress.

- Improve self-awareness.
- Improve self-control.
- Improve attention.

Operational Definitions

Hatha Yoga

The practice of yoga and yogic meditation corresponds in several areas to what we know about the psychology of flow. For instance, Csikszentmihalyi (1990) writes that flow becomes more accessible when one learns control over the body and its senses. In regard to control over the body and its experiences, there are few practices that are older and more efficient than Hatha Yoga. Hatha Yoga is a physical and mental practice designed to unite the mind and body, and there is growing evidence to suggest that the practice of yoga may benefit positive psychological functioning through the implementation of mindfulness and emotional regulation (Franked, Gootjes, Van Strien, 2011, p. 92). Emotional regulation refers to the ability to control and influence the emotions we feel, when we feel them, and how we experience and express them (Gross, 1998).

Yoga has been used to find ease in the body, quiet the mind, and build confidence and awareness in the body for approximately 5,000 years (Serline et, al., 20017). Most forms of yoga practiced in the West can be classified as Hatha Yoga. Hatha practices are designed to invigorate the body and mind in preparation for meditation. Hatha Yoga creates balance, physically and emotionally, through the use of strenuous physical postures, or asanas, combined with breathing techniques, or pranayama. Meditation and guided imagery not only support the physical and emotional achievements of the postures and breathing, they also promote self-actualization, creating a union of the mind, body, and spirit (Gimbel, 1998). Research has shown that yoga can help regulate and calm emotions, reduce stress and improve the mind-body connection (Serline et, al., 20017).

Although yoga has been shown to be a viable technique for improving the performance of the mind and body, little attention has been directed to studying the relationship between yoga and the psychological states of creative flow and mindfulness. (Ahmed, Butzer, Khalsa, 2015). This study suggests that using art therapy interventions, immediately following a yoga practice can benefit the creative process and allow individuals to more fully connect to their minds and bodies.

The Mind-Body Connection

Mind-body health is the discipline that examines the relationship between the brain, mind, and body, specifically involving behavior. The goal is to reduce stress, physical disease and ailments through techniques that direct mental processes. Mind-body medicine is most commonly used for anxiety/depression and for musculoskeletal and myofascial pain syndromes (Butzer, Ahmed & Khalsa, 2016).

There are a number of modalities under the umbrella of mind/body medicine, including relaxation techniques, guided imagery, tai chi, qigong, yoga, and meditation. These techniques can be used in conjunction with conventional medicine or independently. The popularity of mind-body health has grown extensively due to its convenience, low cost and minimal side effects, and most who practice mind-body procedures report feeling positive changes (Butzer, Ahmed & Khalsa, 2016). Hatha Yoga and meditation are ancient mind-body practices that have been used throughout history as self-care and healing modalities. More and more these techniques are becoming established, scientifically recognized practices that are altering the healthcare model and improving lives across the globe (Serline et, al., 20017).

Mindfulness

Mindful meditative practices have long been associated with Eastern traditions such as Yoga and Buddhism. Mindfulness is an attribute of consciousness believed to promote well-being and there is a growing body of research to support its efficacy. Attributes of mindfulness include enhanced mental functioning, self-regulated behavior and positive emotional states (Brown & Ryan, 2003). These practices involve giving your attention to only one thing, either as a religious activity or as a way of becoming calm and relaxed (Serline, et al,. 2007). Both mindfulness and positive psychological principles are being implemented in hospitals, clinics and schools across the nation, and are becoming recognized as strongly correlated to positive emotions and overall well-being.

Emotional Regulation

Emotional regulation refers to the extrinsic and intrinsic processes responsible for monitoring, evaluating, and modifying emotional reactions (Thompson, 1991). These techniques vary depending on culture, but there is one common belief: individuals need to exert some measure of control over their emotions. Nowhere is this dominating sentiment stronger than in the West. One of the central tenets of Western philosophy is the antagonism of reason and emotion (Gross, 1998). However, in recent decades, a new chapter has opened in the discussion of emotional regulation and psychological research has expanded with the emergence of mindfulness.

Researchers and clinicians have shown that mindfulness training can improve emotional disorders, negative mood and reduce physiological responses such as skin conductance and amygdala activity. These findings point to the emotional regulatory function of mindfulness for which recent studies have provided direct experimental evidence (Grecucci, Pappaianni,

Siugzdaite, Theuninck, Job, 2015). Although there is a growing body of research to support the value of mindfulness for the purposes of emotional regulation, the investigation is still in its infancy. There is much to learn about the extent and processes through which mindfulness practices improve emotional regulation (Hill & Updegraff, 2012).

Flow

Mihaly Csikszentmihalyi, a pioneer of modern day creativity research defines creativity as "… any act, idea or product that changes an existing domain, or that transforms an existing domain into a new one" (Csikszentmihalyi, 1996, p. 28). Creativity is unique in that it is accompanied by a feeling of absorption that comes from being in a state that he calls *flow*. Many art therapists have observed how art making in art therapy can promote a state of flow, which in turn can have a therapeutic effect (Chilton & Wilkinson, 2009). In positive psychology, flow, frequently referred to as the zone, is a mental process in which a person performing an activity becomes fully engaged in a feeling of energized concentration, full connection, and enjoyment. In essence, flow is characterized by complete absorption in the activity at hand and accompanied by feelings of being fully present, awake, and alive (Csikszentmihalyi, 1990).

There are many barriers to successfully channeling flow. Cognitive psychologist and a leading creativity researcher, Mark Runco, reported that there are five obstacles that prevent people from acting creatively: learned habits, rules and traditions, perceptual barriers, cultural barriers and emotional barriers. In his study (2011) he argues that all of these potential blocks must be taken into consideration in order to effectively harness flow (Runco & Pritzker, 2011). Despite new developments in creativity and mind-body research, little has been written on methods for intentionally entering and maintaining the flow state.

Positive Psychology

Positive Psychology represents a major paradigm shift in the field of psychology with its major focus involving the study of positive emotions, human character (traits and virtues), and positive institutions (Seligman 2002). In his revised version of the well-being theory, Martin Seligman (2011) introduced the PERMA model, which summarizes five pillars of well-being: positive emotions, engagement, relationships, meaning and accomplishment). The PERMA model connects engagement with the flow state, a construct originally introduced by Mihalyi Csikszentmihalyi (1990) and that refers to "a very rewarding and enjoyable psychological state in which an individual is completely immersed in an activity such that no attention or psychic energy is left for any distractions" Csikszentmihalyi (1990, p2).

Art Therapy

Although creative arts have been used as a tool to enhance aspects of human life for over 40,000 years, the field of art therapy did not emerge until the early 1940's. Art Therapy as a mental health service is being used to promote wellness and prevention in a wide variety of settings nationwide. Art therapy uses art as a means of symbolic communication and expresses personality, emotions and other aspects of human experience. It uses the creative process of art making to improve and enhance the physical, mental, and emotional well-being of individuals of all ages (AATA website).

Yoga and mindfulness are complementary approaches that allow individuals to access the mind-body connection (Serlin et al., 2007). Positive psychology can further complement these approaches by increasing positive emotions and well-being and encourage flow states. Art therapy is the application of the arts and the creative process to support, maintain, and improve the psychosocial, physical, cognitive and spiritual health of individuals. The inclusive nature of this study is based on current and emerging research that art making is a health-enhancing practice and that the integration of these approaches can positively impact the quality of life.

Carl Jung and Mandalas

Carl Jung, the Swiss psychiatrist, is credited with bringing the mandala into Western culture. Traditionally used as a tool for devotion in Eastern Religions, Jung explored the psychological effects and meanings of mandalas. Jung saw mandalas as symbolic of the inner process by which individuals grow toward fulfilling their potential for wholeness. In his writings on mandala symbolism, Carl Jung refers to the mandala as "the psychological expression of the totality of the self" (Henderson, Mascaro & Rosen, 2007). In the mandalas, Jung saw a natural process of generating and resolving inner conflicts that brings about greater complexity, harmony, and stability in the personality. He theorized that the creation of mandalas promotes the process of psychic integration, bringing to the surface themes from the unconscious mind and inner symbols to conscious awareness (Henderson, Mascaro & Rosen, 2007).

Chapter II

Literature Review

Introduction

In the following literature review, the student researcher examined relevant and current information regarding trends in the field. It is an investigation into the connection between Hatha Yoga and Flow Theory. The efficacy of Hatha Yoga is evaluated in conjunction with the literature regarding the mind-body connection, mindfulness techniques, and emotional regulation. Flow Theory is then explored through studies on body movement, positive psychological approaches to well-being and the field of art therapy. This chapter will expand upon the definitions reported in the previous chapter in an effort to concentrate the information, and to better understand how yoga may impact perceived creativity.

Hatha Yoga

Yoga is a physical, mental, and spiritual practice that denotes a variety of schools, practices and goals (White, 2011). Yoga is an ancient practice that developed in India about 5,000 years ago and is considered the embodiment of mind-body medicine (Serline et, al., 2017). The practice aims to integrate the mind, body and breath and was designed to bring balance and health to the physical, mental, emotional and spiritual dimensions of an individual (Kraftsow, 1999). In a recent study, the number of yoga practitioners in America increased by fifty percent to over thirty six million practitioners (Yoga Journal, 2016).

The primary type of yoga practiced in the United States comes from the branch of Hatha Yoga, which is known for its physically demanding postures (asana) and breath control (pranayama). The word hatha can be translated two ways: as “willful/forceful”, or the yoga of activity, and as “sun” (ha) and “moon” (tha), the yoga of balance (Serline et, al., 2017). Hatha practices are designed to establish balance in the body in preparation for meditation. Hatha practitioners and researchers claim a number of health benefits from practicing yoga. The physical benefits include increased flexibility and balance, enhanced immune function, and increased blood flow, a lower risk of hypertension, diabetes and cardiac conditions. The psychological benefits include reductions of stress, anxiety, depression, eating disorders, phobias and addiction, as well as relaxation, focused attention, increase in self-esteem and self-awareness (Serline et, al., 20017).

Yoga is believed to enhance healing and reduce stress by decreasing the fight-or-flight activity of the sympathetic nervous system and increase the parasympathetic nervous system response of rest, relaxation and repair. When the sympathetic nervous system components of the brain are activated, it produces a "cascade of physiological, behavioral and psychological effects" (Ross & Thomas, 2010, p.3). It is believed that the continual stimulation of the sympathetic nervous system is the primary contributor to diseases such as autoimmune disorders, obesity, substance abuse, diabetes and cardiovascular disease (Ross & Thomas, 2010).

Research from Boston University, New York Medical College and Columbia University have proposed a theory for why yoga has such a profound effect on the autonomic nervous system. The theory suggests that the techniques involved in yoga stimulate a nerve that is responsible for restoring optimal functioning or homeostasis. This particular area in the body is called the vagus nerve and is often referred to as the pathway to the parasympathetic nervous system. These researchers suggest that yoga may be one of the most effective tools available for managing stress and stress related diseases in adults, adolescents and children (Streeter, Gerbarg, Saper, Ciraulo, & Brown, 2011).

Although yoga has been shown to be a viable technique for improving the performance of the mind and body, little attention has been directed to studying the relationship between yoga and the psychological states of flow and mindfulness. In a longitudinal study (2016) musicians enrolled in a 2-month fellowship program in 2005, 2006 and 2007 were invited to participate in a yoga and meditation series. Fellows not participating in the yoga program were recruited separately as a control group. All participants completed baseline and end program questionnaires evaluating dispositional flow, mindfulness, confusion, and music performance anxiety. When compared to the control groups, yoga participants reported significant decreases in confusion and increases in dispositional flow. Yoga participants in the 2006 sample also reported significant increases in the mindfulness subscale of awareness. Correlational analyses revealed that increases in participants' dispositional flow and mindfulness were associated with decreases in confusion and music performance anxiety. This study demonstrates the commonalities between positive psychology and yoga, both of which are focused on enhancing human performance and promoting beneficial psychological states. The results suggest that yoga and meditation may enhance the states of flow and mindful awareness, and reduce confusion (Butzer, Ahmed, Khalsa, 2016).

The Mind-body Connection

For centuries Western society believed in the separation of mind and body. The mind was seen as superior to the body because it was viewed as the center of reason, identity and spirituality while the body was seen as home to untamed emotions and primal urges. However, as the filed of neurology developed it proved that the mind and body are inextricably linked, and that the relationship can exert a positive or negative influence on well-being and creativity (Miller, 2016).

Walter Bradford Cannon, the Harvard physiologist that coined the term "fight or flight response," proved that emotions affect body chemistry, heart rate and the activity of every cell and organ in the body (Brown & Fee, 2002). Cannon studied the human body's automatic response to strong emotion. He observed five primary bodily reactions to intense stimuli which constitute the fight or flight response: muscle tension, flooding of hormones, the altering of blood sugar levels, the redistribution of blood, and the limiting of higher-level functions in the brain. Cannon concluded that the regions of the brain associated with executive decision-making and goal-directed behaviors were heavily impacted, making humans less productive and cognitively predisposed to repeat the same actions over and over again while under stress (Brown & Fee, 2002). Cannon's conclusions address the impact of stress on flow and support the claim that a reduction in stress could benefit creative states.

Recent dialogue between Western and Eastern traditions has stimulated exploration of the relationship between mind and body and their impact on the creative process. More specifically, scientists have begun asking how physical activity impacts cognition. In a study conducted at Stanford University (2014) researchers ran a series of experiments that looked at the positive effects of body movement on creative ideation in forty adult, university students. The design of the experiments consisted of two subject groups: indoor vs. dynamic outdoors and sitting vs. walking. The design had four conditions of sitting inside, walking on a treadmill inside, sitting in a moving wheelchair outside and walking outside. After receiving task instructions, participants heard three prompts and had five minutes to generate analogies for all three (Oppexxo & Schwartx, 2014).

Of those who walked, 95% generated at least one novel, high-quality analogy compared with the 50% of those who sat. The results of the study demonstrated that walking substantially enhanced 81% of participants' creativity. Walking led to an increase in analogical creativity, and walking outside produced the most novel and high quality analogies and ideas. In the discussion of the study the researchers asked, "would other forms of mild physical activity have a similar elevating effects?" The explanation they provided was that "…it may be the mind-freeing quality of engaging in a comfortable task (e.g. knitting) rather than exercise" (Oppexxo & Schwartx, p. 1148).

Although the differences between walking and yoga may seem extensive, many of their principles are the same. Unlike a traditional workout, walking and yoga both focus on precise body movements that allow us to slowly transition from one position to the next. They are both low-impact, physical activities that promote circulation, and help clear the mind. Moreover, these specific practices have few adverse side effects, and have been shown to lower stress levels and increase physical and emotional well-being (Ross & Thomas, 2010).

Broad ranges of mind-body therapies (MBTs) are being used in public health today, and a growing body of clinical science research has resulted in evidence-based integration of many MBTs into clinical practice. Research has identified some of the physiological correlates of MBT practices, leading to a better understanding of the processes by which emotional, cognitive and psychosocial factors can influence health and well-being. In particular, genomics and neuroimaging results describe some of the processes involved in the mind-body connection and the consequences that they have on health (Muehsam, et al., 2017).

In a review on functional genomic and neurological correlates of mind-body therapies (2017), researchers from University of California, San Diego examined the correlates of MBTs. The studies showed that individuals who participated in MBTs exhibited changes in sympathetic nervous system activation. The primary factors involved were associated with immune function, inflammation, and neural function. These components are predominantly relevant for attention, learning, and emotional regulation. Although the review had limitations, including broad diversity of study designs being examined and MBTs being studied, the data generated by these studies has contributed significantly towards a better understanding of the biological mechanisms underlying MBTs. This understanding may in turn guide mental health approaches in the future and promote more inclusive methodologies that emphasize care for the whole person (Muehsam, et al., 2017).

The Practice of Mindfulness

Mindfulness is the psychological process of bringing one's attention to experiences occurring in the present moment. This method is continually being implemented in both medical and psychology fields and is believed to integrate mind and body and promote and maintain overall well-being in practitioners (Serlinet, al., 2007). Mindfulness is considered a learned skill that has been adopted by multiple psychological orientations including dialectical behavioral therapy, mindfulness-based cognitive therapy and acceptance commitment therapy (Corey, 2009). In addition many medical hospitals and clinics are implementing mindfulness techniques as complementary approaches to more conventional interventions (Serlinet, al., 2007).

According to mindfulness research review done by Jeffery Greeson (2008, p.1), "there is rapidly accumulating evidence in the field of complementary health practices that greater mindfulness can not only reduce stress and stress related medical symptoms but can also enhance positive emotions and quality of life." Greeson concludes that adults who participate in mindfulness research consistently report less stress, anxiety and depressive symptoms and report more overall joyfulness, inspiration, gratitude, hopefulness, contentment, vitality and satisfaction with life. Adult studies also conclude that mindfulness-based practices can improve pain and addiction and can increase self-esteem, coping skills, energy, enthusiasm for life and the ability to relax (Greeson, 2008).

Goodman, Kashdan, Mallard, and Schumann, (2014) examined the effectiveness of "mindfulness-based exercises" with adult college athletes. In the five-week study, participants attended eight ninety-minute group intervention sessions that consisted of Hatha Yoga, breathing meditations, body scans and visualization practices. Participants completed self-reported measures before and after the mindfulness interventions. The themes that were measured included: mindfulness, tolerance and negative affect, avoidance, goal motivation, perceived stress, commitment to values, cognitive diffusion, and psychological distress. The study had several limitations including a small sample size and lack of diverse ethnicities and socioeconomic backgrounds. However, the results revealed participants with high levels of anxiety at pre-test had significant reduction in anxiety symptoms three months after completing the intervention. According to the research the participants reported "...greater mindfulness, greater goal-directed energy, and less perceived stress than before the investigation. Participants also reported greater tolerance of negative experiences such that participants reported greater comfort with disgust and anxiety after the intervention" (Goodman, Kashdan, Mallard, & Schumann, 2014).

Many of these cross-cultural, mind-body discourses have proven productive in identifying more adaptive forms of embodiment. Studies suggest that there are two key constructs in mind-body approaches and they are dispositional mindfulness (DM) and interoceptive awareness (IA). Dispositional mindfulness is defined by someone's awareness and attention to what they are thinking and feeling, and interoceptive awareness refers to the perception of internal bodily sensations (Hanley, Mehling & Garland, 2017). In a study done by University of Utah, Center on Mindfulness and Integrative Health Development and University of California, San Francisco Medical Center (Hanley, Mehling & Garland, 2017), researchers explored the relationship between scores on measures of IA and DM. The study examined the networks of association between IA and DM in adults and aimed at addressing the relationship between these constructs and well-being. The researchers concluded that IA and DM were tightly interwoven, partly overlapping constructs. Greater DM was strongly linked to greater IA. Additionally, both IA and DM appear to be independently associated with enhanced psychological well-being (Hanley, Mehling & Garland, 2017).

Control of the Senses: Emotional Regulation

Discovering and promoting ways that help regulate emotions has been a recurrent concern in the field of psychology, given that how one feels and reacts to and expresses emotions can have both short and long term effects on physical and mental health. In a systematic review of studies by the Brazilian Institute of Neuroscience (2015) researchers examined the effects of yoga on emotional variables to better understand the relationship between yoga and emotional regulation (Dalpiaz, et. al, 2015). The review examined the primary psychological outcomes of yoga and their physiological correlates in healthy sample studies. The results of these studies demonstrated that yoga increased positive affect, positive mood, anger control, resiliency and well-being. Yoga was shown to reduce stress, anxiety, verbal aggression and symptoms of depression. Finally, the researchers concluded that yoga might foster emotional regulation skills through such mechanisms as reappraisal, attention regulation, self-monitoring, self-awareness, and autonomic regulation (Dalpiaz, et. al, 2015). These studies suggest that yoga may help maintain a state of physical and mental balance and increase overall well-being in individuals.

In a similar study (2011) done by the Institute of Psychology at the University of Rotterdam, researchers examined the neurophysiological correlates of cognitive reappraisal in practitioners of a yogic meditation program. Reappraisal is believed to involve the interaction of multiple cognitive processes, such as attention, memory and imagery. A key aspect of many meditative practices is how to maintain a peaceful mind throughout positive and negative life events. The program involved several tools including meditation, breathing techniques, and cognitive coping strategies such as reappraisal that helped practitioners regulate their emotions. Twenty-four healthy participants took part in the study and they were recruited at random among undergraduate students (Gootjes, Franken & Van Strien, 2011).

The yogic group consisted of 12 individuals and their practices ranged from daily to three times a week, ranging from twenty to sixty minutes per session. The control group consisted of twelve individuals and had no prior experience with any form of meditation. The participants' positive and negative affect was assessed as well as their ability to control thoughts. Individuals underwent a series of tasks while the researchers mapped the electrodes neurologically. The results were that the yogic group scored significantly higher on positive affect and their ability to control thoughts over the control group (Gootjes, Franken & Van Strien, 2011). The findings support that yoga and meditation can improve multiple cognitive processes, such as attention, memory, concentration and imagery.

Martin Levine, a Harvard researcher and theorist in cognitive-experimental psychology, explored the similarities between Buddhism, Yoga and Positive Psychology. In his book (2009)

Levine argues that recent developments in mental health approaches suggest that the field is becoming more and more influenced by Eastern philosophies such as Buddhism and Yoga. The author highlights six comparisons: 1. They are concerned with alleviating inner suffering. 2. They are humanistic and naturalistic. 3. They see the human being as being caught in a causal framework, in a matrix of forces that consists of cravings and drives. 4. They teach compassion, concern, and unconditional positive regard toward all beings. 5. They share the ideal of maturing and growth. 6. They acknowledge that the mind functions both a superficial as well as a deeper level.

The principal thesis of his research is that Buddhist and Yogic practices may provide unique access to mental functioning, giving rise to metacognition and to self-reflection. It is in this vein that Levine offers a blend of Western science and Eastern practices to help individuals monitor thoughts and regulate emotions. The goal is to become more peaceful and less anxious, an objective he calls "mature happiness" (Levine, 2009, p.59). Levine encourages mental health professionals to explore these approaches as they may provide answers to questions regarding self-transformation and improvements in quality of life (Levine, 2009).

Flow Theory

In positive psychology, flow is a mental state of operation in which a person performing an activity becomes fully immersed in a feeling of energized focus, full involvement, and enjoyment in the process or activity. Flow is characterized by complete absorption in what one does, and a resulting loss in one's sense of space and time. The primary expert on flow theory is Hungarian psychologist Mihaly Csikszentmihalyi. Csikszentmihalyi first introduced the concept of flow in his book 'Flow: The Psychology of Optimal Experience' where he describes it as the "optimal experience" (Csikszentmihalyi, 1990, p.5). He called it flow because so many of the artists he interviewed used the metaphor of a current of water to describe their optimal experience. Thousands of interviews have identified the flow experience in people of varying ages and types and across diverse cultures. However, flow is not a modern concept. *Being one with the flow* of life is a millennia-old teaching that appears in Christian mystic, contemplative, yogic, Taoist, Buddhist, Islamic, Jewish, and other spiritual traditions (Csikszentmihalyi, 1990).

The spontaneous outpouring of joy surrounding flow can be related to *ecstasy,* which in the original Greek "ekstasis" means, "to stand beside" ordinary experience and to step into an altered state of consciousness (Harper, 2017). Achieving this experience is considered to be personal and depends on the ability of the individual. According to Csikszentmihályi, one's desire to overcome challenges in order to achieve their goals not only leads to optimal experiences, but to a greater sense of well-being and overall satisfaction with life (Csikszentmihalyi, 1997).

A flow state can be entered while performing any activity, although it is most likely to occur when one is wholeheartedly performing a task or activity for intrinsic purposes. Csikszentmihalyi describes the flow as being "autotelic" or having an end or purpose in itself (Csikszentmihalyi, 1990, p.67). The term autotelic derives from two Greek words, *auto* meaning self and *telos* meaning goal (Csikszentmihalyi, 1990, p.67). The more passive the activity the less likely it is to elicit the autotelic and in turn the flow experience. While the activities that induce flow vary greatly and are multifaceted, Csikszentmihályi asserts that the experience of flow is similar despite the action (Csikszentmihayli, 2000).

Flow theory postulates three conditions that must be met to achieve a flow state. The first is that an individual must be involved in an activity with a clear set of goals and progress. This adds direction and structure to the task. The second condition is the task at hand must have clear and immediate feedback. This assists the person in negotiating any changing demands and allows them to adjust their performance to maintain flow. The third condition is that one must achieve a balance between the perceived challenges of the task at hand and their own perceived skills. Confidence is necessary to one's ability to complete the task at hand (Csikszentmihalyi, 1997).

A primary feature of flow is the balance between difficulty and skill. For example, if the task being undertaken is too difficult or too easy flow cannot be reached. To achieve the optimal experience a balance must be struck between the challenge of the task and the skill of the performer. Csikszentmihalyi explains that both skill level and challenge must be matched in order for intrinsic motivations to induce the sensation of full immersion in the activity (Csikszentmihalyi, 1990). In a study of flow theory and research (2001) Csíkszentmihályi joined with Dr. Jeanne Nakamura to identify six factors that encompass a flow experience. These factors include: intense and focused concentration, merging of action and awareness, loss of self consciousness, a sense of personal control or agency over the situation or activity, distortion of temporal experience, intrinsically rewarding (Nakamura & Csikszentmihalyi, 2001). These qualities can appear independently of each other, but only in combination do they constitute a so-called flow experience.

The Body In Flow

Most people are aware of the importance of health and physical fitness, but the almost unlimited potential for enjoyment that the body offers often remains unexploited (Csikszentmihalyi, 1990). In Mihalyi Csikszentmihalyi's leading flow research (1990) he states the following:

> Everything the body can do is potentially enjoyable. Yet many people ignore this capacity, and use their physical equipment as little as possible, leaving its ability

> to provide flow unexploited. When left undeveloped, the senses give us chaotic information… If the functions of the body are left to atrophy, the quality of life becomes merely adequate, and for some even dismal. But if one takes control of what the body can do, and learns to impose order on physical sensations, entropy yields to a sense of harmony in consciousness. (p. 95).

Due to the accessibility of physical movements and activities, Csikszentmihalyi argues that the body provides an ideal opportunity for initiating flow states and improving quality of life. The key component is learning to control the body and its senses (Csikszentmihalyi, 1990).

Correlational studies (Butzer, Ahmed, Khalsa, 2016) have demonstrated the commonalities between positive psychology and yoga, both of which are focused on enhancing human performance and promoting beneficial psychological states. Research in this area is continuing to grow, but early investigations suggest that yoga and meditation may enhance the states of flow and mindful awareness, through control of the senses (Butzer, Ahmed, Khalsa, 2016). In his first study, Csikszentmihalyi (1990) explains that because physical activities are so easily accessible, they are among the easiest steps one can take toward improving happiness and creativity. He claims that flow becomes more readily available when one begins to learn control over the body and its senses. Csikszentmihalyi writes, “Of all the great Eastern methods for training the body, one of the oldest and most diffuse is the set of practices known as Hatha Yoga” (Csikszentmihalyi, 1990, p.103-104). The word “yoga” comes from the root, “yuj” (meaning “unity” or “yoke”), indicating that the purpose of yoga is to unite the mind and body, and to bring individuals closer to their highest nature. From here Csikszentmihalyi outlines the eight limbs of yoga and explains that each step involves building up increasingly higher levels of skill in controlling consciousness. He argues that the similarities between yoga and flow are extremely strong, in part because "both try to achieve a joyous, self-forgetful involvement through concentration, which in turn is made possible by a discipline of the body" (Csikszentmihalyi, 1990, p.105).

In a study by Briegel-Jones, Eubank and Knowles (2013), researchers examined the effects of a yoga practice on mindfulness and flow in elite youth swimmers. The study investigated the direct effects of yoga on creative flow. The aim of this study was to explore in detail the subjective experiences regarding the perceived effects of yoga. The researchers performed a ten-week long yoga intervention on mindfulness and dispositional flow. The study was a mixed methods design where both qualitative and quantitative data was collected. Participants were chosen from national training sites and given two questionnaires as well as the Dispositional Flow Short Scale 2 (DFS-2) (Briegel-Jones, Eubank, & Knowles, 2013).

The qualitative data suggested that the ten-week yoga intervention had a positive impact on a range of physiological, cognitive and performance parameters that included elements of mindfulness and flow. The researchers claimed "There was evidence of participants acting with greater awareness when engaged in an activity, including swimming training and competition. Although not taught per se within the yoga program, participants also reported improvements in the ability to reframe negative thoughts through the application of the yoga relaxation techniques. In addition, improvements in flow disposition dimensions were suggested including enhanced concentration and greater sense of control when involved both in swimming and also that these has transferred to that of school related activities" (Briegel-Jones, Eubank, & Knowles, 2013).

The similarities between yoga and flow are extremely strong. However, many critics prefer to stress the differences between flow and yoga. Their main difference is that, whereas flow attempts to fortify the self, the goal of yoga and many other Eastern techniques is to eliminate it. According to yogic philosophy, Samadhi is the last stage before entering Nirvana, where the individual self is said to merge with the universal consciousness. Therefore it could be argued that yoga and flow tend toward diametrically opposing outcomes (Csikszentmihalyi, 1990).

Positive Psychology Approach to Well-Being and Creativity

Positive psychology is the scientific study of positive human functioning and flourishing on multiple levels that include the biological, personal, relational, institutional, cultural, and global dimensions of life (Seligman, Csikszentmihalyi, 2000). From a positive psychology approach there is less emphasis on diagnosis and pathology and more on the promotion and maintenance of psychological well-being. Martin Seligman, the founder of positive psychology advises mental health professionals to shift their goals from "understanding misery and undoing the disabling conditions of life to exploring what makes life worth living and building the enabling conditions of a life worth living" (Seligman, 2011, p.2).

The primary question of positive psychology is: What makes life most worth living? Originally Martin Seligman identified three primary components that contribute to happiness: "positive emotion" or maximizing pleasurable experiences in life, "engagement" or being in a state of flow, and "meaning" or belonging and or serving something you believe to be greater than the self (Seligman, 2011 p.2). As his research continued Seligman developed two other elements: "accomplishment" or pursuing success and developing and maintaining "positive relationships" (Seligman, 2011 p.2). According to Seligman and Csikszentmihalyi, the central concerns of positive psychology are centered on three issues: positive emotions, positive individual traits, and positive institutions. Positive emotions refer to being content with the past, happy in the present and hopeful for the future. Positive individual traits focus on individual strengths and virtues. Finally, positive institutions refer to families, schools, businesses and societies that foster better communities by encouraging justice, responsibility, nurturance, teamwork and tolerance. They are based on collective strengths and methods of enhancing communities (Seligman & Csikszentmihalyi, 2000).

From a scientific standpoint, researchers have only recently begun to focus on measuring positive psychology constructs such as life satisfaction, well-being and creativity. In a study conducted by University of Ohio Psychology Department, researchers investigated the impact of positive and negative affect on creativity (Charyton, et al., 2009). The quasi-experimental study hypothesized that optimism would enhance creative flow. Data on creativity, optimism, and pessimism, positive and negative affect, and current and usual happiness ratings were collected on 161 college students enrolled in an introductory psychology class. Participants were tested using a demographic questionnaire, a happiness scale, and five assessments used to measure creativity and positive and negative affect (Charyton, et al., 2009).

The findings indicated that both positive and negative affect contributed to creative characteristics. Contrary to literature emphasizing positive affect, characteristics of positive and negative affect were related to increased scores in creativity. Although some negative emotions detracted from creativity, they found that others contributed to higher scoring. For example, two negative mood states (scared and nervous) decreased participants' creativity scores. However, those who reported feeling distressed and guilty demonstrated more creative characteristics. Likewise, pessimism enhanced creativity but optimism did not have a significant effect. The study concluded that positive affect did not significantly impede creative flow—interest, strength, and usual happiness all contributed and were found to predict higher levels of creative ideation. Furthermore, heightened anxiety and fear were the two emotions that were found to be the most harmful to creativity (Charyton, et al., 2009).

In another study conducted by the Swarthmore College and the Positive Psychology Center at the University of Pennsylvania, researchers conducted a two year study that examined if character strengths can predict future well-being in adolescents (Gillham et al,. 2001). Although the study had limitations including small sample size and lack of racial diversity, the researchers discovered other-directed and transcendence strengths can predict well-being (Gillham et al,. 2001). Participants that displayed "other-directed strengths such as teamwork, forgiveness and kindness predicted fewer symptoms of depression" and those with "transcendence strengths such as hope, gratitude and meaning in life predicted greater overall life satisfaction" (Gillham et al,. 2001, p.31). The study concluded that character strengths that build relationships and purpose predict future well-being (Gillham et al,. 2001).

Flow in Art Therapy

Art Therapy is a mental health service that promotes "wellness and prevention in a wide variety of settings including hospitals, psychiatric and rehabilitation facilities, wellness centers, forensic institutions, schools, crisis centers, senior communities, private practice, and other clinical and community settings" (AATA, website). The American Art Therapy Association (2012) defines art therapy as "a mental health profession that uses the creative process of art making to improve and enhance the physical, mental, and emotional well-being of individuals of all ages" (AATA website).

Lynn Kapitan, Professor and Director of the Art Therapy Doctoral Program at Mount Mary University, began researching flow in art therapy in 2004. In her phenomenological study (2004) Kapitan observed disenchantment in the workplace of art therapists. She was exploring what factors contributed to burnout and why art therapists found it difficult to maintain their own art practices. Her search for data led her into the terrain of the "toxic" work environment, which each of the study's participants in separate interviews depicted as "barren and devoid of clear, flowing water" (Kapitan, 2004, p.54-55). Kapitan described the interviews saying "Whether draining away, becoming polluted, or evaporating into cracked, lifeless soil, the imagery accumulated of desperately desired, life-giving water to quench the participants' creative thirst" (Kapitan, 2004, p.54-55). Later when the participants were asked to reimagine how their work lives might be different, each art therapist depicted similar transformations from feeling cut off to being one with an abundant flow of life energy (Kapitan, 2004).

Kapitan's (2004) results led her to conclude that flow can set up conditions for developing high concentration, increased self-esteem, and greater health and well-being. Kapitan argues that because flow has been theoretically and empirically linked to creativity and improved well-being, the study of flow should be of particular interest to the field of art therapy. She writes "Art therapists may facilitate personal growth by helping individuals enter and maintain a state of flow in their art making" (Kapitan, 2013, p.66). In particular she believes that flow is an active ingredient in art therapy's efficacy, and its potential to relieve debilitative anxiety.

Similarly to Lynn Kapitan, authors Wilkinson and Chilton (2013) argue that positive psychology has much to offer the field of art therapy, which in turn is uniquely poised to contribute to the study of optimal functioning. Their article 'Positive Art Therapy: Linking Positive Psychology to Art Therapy Theory, Practice and Research' discusses the relationship of positive psychology to art therapy and its capacity to mobilize client strengths, induce experiences of flow and positive emotions. The disease model has not advanced psychology closer to the prevention of mental illnesses, and these authors argue that identifying and building on human strengths does more to develop resilience against psychiatric problems and future stressors (Wilkinson & Chilton, 2013).

Positive psychologists suggest that flow is enhanced when people are able to engage in their highest faculties or "signature strengths" (Wilkinson & Chilton, 2013). Art therapy often has been associated with identifying and capitalizing on client strengths. The authors explain that art therapy assessments could be greatly enhanced were therapist able to develop or modify instruments that correspond to existing psychological tests of strengths. In doing so, clearer criteria could be established for emphasizing client strengths that uniquely emerge in the art therapy process. With respect to the paradigm shift toward positive psychology, Wilkinson and Chilton called attention to the unique benefits of the art therapy process to generate mastery and flow, to improve mood, and to inspire, create, and illuminate meaning. This view emphasizes the claim that art therapy should be used as a method to encourage creative flow, improved cognitive function and overall well-being.

Summary

The present study strived to provide the field of art therapy with the most relevant literature regarding yoga and creativity research. The purpose of the literature review was to collect information regarding the efficacy of using yoga to initiate flow as a means of facilitating personal growth through art therapy. Art therapists have long upheld the benefits of self-expression as well as the use of art to uncover unconscious knowledge. As Kaplan (2000) explained, "when art making partakes of the characteristics of 'flow,' it provides the kind of optimal experience that produces feelings of psychological growth and makes life in general more worth living" (Kaplan, 2000, p. 76). From this literature yoga was found to be correlated with flow states, and in turn flow was theoretically and empirically linked to creativity and improved well-being. Therefore, the connection between yoga and flow may be of particular interest to the field of art therapy. In summary, the researcher sought to answer the call made by J.P. Guilford, and to explore how yoga might impact individual creativity and in turn perceived levels of stress and well-being.

Chapter III

Methodology

This section describes the investigative focus, research methodology, and specific methods used in the study. The methodology used was a mixed method research framework implementing both qualitative and quantitative data collection. The researcher explains how the necessary data and information to address the research objectives and questions was collected, presented and analyzed. Hypotheses and research questions, research design, measurement instruments, data sources, collection techniques and analysis are provided. This section also explains the design and construction of the hatha yoga and mandala art intervention.

Hypotheses and Research Questions

The first hypothesis for this study was that integrating the principles of positive psychology and mindfulness, alongside a practice of Hatha Yoga would have an affect on the creative process. The secondary hypothesis was that the act of practicing yoga and meditation, combined with the art directives would be beneficial to strengthening the mind-body connection and improving overall well-being in participants, as well as aid in stress reduction. Additionally, the research sought to answer the following questions:

1. Is there a relationship between body movement work and creativity?
2. What is the impact of yoga on health and well-being?
3. Is change observable in the artwork or in body sensations after a designated routine of yoga and art?

Research Design

This research design was a mixed method design combining quantitative and qualitative components. The quantitative component was a quasi-experimental design that included a demographic survey and a pre-test/post-test creativity questionnaire. The pre and post-tests were used to measure participants' creativity styles prior to and after participation in the three meeting group intervention. The qualitative components included self-report journal inventories that the participants completed at the end of each meeting.

Measures

The *Demographics Survey* (Appendix F) was used to collect information about the participants' gender, age, ethnicity, marital status, education, and employment status. The demographic information was collected prior to the experiment. Quantitative data was collected using a self-report inventory called the *Creativity Styles Questionnaire-Revised* (CSQ-R) (Appendix A). The purpose of the questionnaire was to see how people go about accomplishing the creative act.

The *CSQ-R* (Appendix A) is a self-report assessment that consists of eight scales that include: Kumar and Holman's Global Measure of Creative Capacity, belief in the unconscious process, use of techniques, use of other people, final product orientation, environmental control/behavioral self-regulation, superstition and the use of the senses. The questionnaire consists of seventy-eight questions and utilizes a likert scale answering system (Kumar, Kemmler & Holman, 1997). The assessment measures beliefs about and strategies for going about being creative. This provided understanding into the specific styles of creativity that were exhibited both before and after participating in the research study. In the past the Creativity Style's Questionnaire has been recorded as a measurement with low internal reliability.

However, the CSQ-R subscales have shown improved reliabilities over the previous CSQ instrument. Recent research has verified the improvements made in the revision and overall the measurement is considered a trusted instrument in the field of creativity research with both high validity and reliability (Kumar et al., 1991).

Additionally, Qualitative data was evaluated through the use of the contemplative journal entries designed by the researcher. Participants were encouraged to discuss their experiences in detail, but there were three mandatory questions:

1. Explain your experience with the yoga and meditation?
2. Do you believe the bodywork had an effect on your creative process? If so, how were you or your art affected?
3. Do you think your practice strengthened your mind-body connection and/or decreased stress levels?

Pre-Screening

Before the study began, the researcher communicated with the prospective participants via phone, email and in person in order to explain the research more specifically, and determine the eligibility of the participants. Eligible participants were adults over the age of eighteen. The researcher described the purpose of the research study, and provided information regarding requirements for the sessions, including location of study, number and length of sessions, time requirement, and consent forms required for participation of the study.

Participants and Recruitment

The researcher recruited adults age eighteen and over. The number of participants for the research was 18 individuals and they were selected by ad correspondence throughout the Lodi,

Stockton and Santa Cruz areas. Social media such as *Facebook* (Appendix C) was used to advertise as well as *Recruitment Fliers* (Appendix D) and word of mouth. Participation in the study was voluntary and participants were given the option to self-assign to either the control group or the experimental group.

Informed Consent

Informed Consent Forms (Appendix G) were provided at the first group meeting explaining the purpose of the study, potential risks and benefits, and confidentiality, including its limitations. The informed consent also explained that participants are able to withdraw from the study at any time without consequence. The consent forms included an artwork release section that allowed the researcher to use questionnaires, tests, artwork and journals provided in the sessions for research purposes.

Location

The intervention and data collection was conducted in three locations, Vinyasa Flow Yoga Studio in Stockton, California (Appendix E), and two private residences located in Lodi, CA and Soquel, CA. Both locations were large studio spaces that fit the groups comfortably and were large enough to practice yoga and create art. Participants sat in large circles on yoga mats for the yoga practice and closing meditations. Art supplies were placed on tables in the back of the room and art making took place on the participants yoga mats post yoga class. The researcher ensured the location was calm and conveniently located for the participants with comfortable seating and available amenities.

Materials

Art Supplies. A variety of art making materials were provided including: white paper with pre-drawn circles for mandalas, various types of construction paper, magazines, scissors, glue sticks, color pencils, oil pastels, watercolor paint, paintbrushes, water cups, painting rags, #2 pencils, ball point pens, erasers and colored markers. A large tarp was used to protect the floor of the studio space. All artwork and journals entries were collected and placed in their individual envelopes after each session.

Yoga Supplies. The yoga materials were supplied by the yoga studio and venue of the research. Each participant was provided with the proper yoga tools, which included yoga mats, straps, blocks, bolsters, eye pillows, two blankets and towels.

Procedure

This study was a three-week long yoga and art therapy intervention program; consisting of three ninety minute sessions that took place once a week during a time that was convenient for the participants. For the experimental group, each session included a half hour Hatha Yoga class, following a ten-minute guided meditation, as well as the mandala art assessment. For the control group, each session included an hour for the mandala art assessment. Below the sessions are listed in detail. Each participant was first assigned a code that was printed on a manila envelope, in order to maintain anonymity. The individual codes on the envelopes were used to contain the participants' demographic information, pre and post-tests, as well as their contemplative journal entries and artwork.

First Meeting/Introduction

During the first meeting/introduction the participants were provided with an overview of the study, and were allowed time for questions and answers. Once the overview was given and any questions were answered, the researcher began the study by distributing the *Informed Consent Forms* (Appendix G), the coded *Demographics Survey* (Appendix F), and the coded pre tests: *CSQ-R* (Appendix A). The researcher then collected the Informed Consent, Demographics Survey, CSQ-R pre-tests and handed out the coded contemplative journals.

The experimental group was instructed through a 30-minute Hatha Yoga class as well as a 10-minute guided mediation at the end of the practice. The participants then partook in the mandala making art experiential, which focused on mindfulness. At the end of the experiential the researcher thoroughly explained the process of the contemplative journal to the participants, and asked them three questions to reflect on as homework:

1. Explain your experience with the yoga and meditation?
2. Do you believe the bodywork had an effect on your creative process? If so, how were you or your art affected?
3. Do you think your practice strengthened your mind-body connection and/or decreased stress levels?

At the end of the course the researcher discussed the next meeting and then the group closed for the day.

The control group did not receive the 30-minute Hatha Yoga class or guided meditation treatment and the participants in this group went straight to the mandala making art experiential after completing the informed consent, demographics surveys, CSQ-R pre-tests. At the end of the art experiential the researcher discussed the next meeting and then the group closed for the day.

Second Meeting

In the second session, the researcher did a check in with the participants from both the experimental and control groups to evaluate potential psychological distress. Next, the experimental groups were instructed through a 30-minute Hatha Yoga class as well as a 10-minute guided mediation at the end of the practice. The participants then partook in the mandala making art experiential, which focused on mindfulness. At the end of the experiential the researcher gave the participants the same three questions to reflect on in their contemplative journals as homework. At the end the researcher discussed the next meeting and then the group will close for the day.

In the second session, the control group did not receive the 30-minute Hatha Yoga class or guided meditation treatment and the participants in this group went straight to the mandala making art experiential. At the end of the art experiential the researcher discussed the next meeting and then the group will close for the day.

Directive: Mandalas

Materials: Paper, magazines, scissors, glue sticks, colored pencils, markers, oil pastels.

The researcher will provide the following questions for the participants to think about while creating their journal entries at their leisure:

1. Explain your experience with the yoga and meditation?
2. Do you believe the bodywork had an effect on your creative process? If so, how were you or your art affected?
3. Do you think your practice strengthened your mind-body connection and/or decreased stress levels?

Third/Final Meeting

In the third session, the researcher did a check in with the participants from both the experimental and control groups to evaluate potential psychological distress. Next, the experimental group was instructed through a 30-minute Hatha Yoga class as well as a 10-minute guided meditation at the end of the practice. The participants then created their final mandalas in the art experiential, which again focused on mindfulness. At the end of the final experiential the researcher gave the participants the same three questions to reflect on in their contemplative journals. The reflection entry took place in session because this was the final meeting. At the end of the reflection period the coded journals were collected and stored in the corresponding manila envelopes.

In the third session, the control group did not receive the 30-minute Hatha Yoga class or guided meditation treatment and the participants in this group went straight to the mandala making art experiential.

The researcher will then administer the post inventory; *CSQ-R* (Appendix A) to both the experimental and control groups, and allowed time for the participants to complete them. The post tests were then collected and stored in the corresponding manila envelops. Once the self-report inventories were completed, the researcher provide the participants with a *debriefing statement* (Appendix I) that provided a formal thank you for participating in the course, as well as a *mental health support information sheet* (Appendix J) that informs them of counseling centers that can provide services if needed.

Directive: Mandalas

Materials: Paper, magazines, scissors, glue sticks, colored pencils, markers, oil pastels.

The researcher provided the following questions for the participants to think about while creating their journal entries at their leisure:

1. Explain your experience with the yoga and meditation?

2. Do you believe the bodywork had an effect on your creative process? If so, how were you or your art affected?

3. Do you think your practice strengthened your mind-body connection and/or decreased stress levels?

Data Collection

This research study used both qualitative and quantitative measures in order to evaluate the value and experience of the participants in the study. *The Demographic Survey* (Appendix F) was given once at the beginning of the study and was used to collect background information on the participants. Next, the pre test, self-report inventories was used to measure the effects of the study in a quantitative capacity. The *CSQ-R* (Appendix A) was be used as a method of gauging the participants' perceptions of their creative styles prior to the study.

After the study, the posttest and self-report inventories were used to measure the effects of the study in a quantitative capacity. The *CSQ-R* (Appendix A) was used as a method of gauging the participants' perceptions of their creative styles after the study. The results taken at the beginning of the experiment were then compared with the results taken at the end, in order to determine if creativity styles were impacted.

Qualitatively, the researcher examined the contemplative journal entries to measure the efficacy of the components for the study. Themes were analyzed based on the participants' answers to the journal questions that were prompted at the end of each session. The researcher then evaluated the qualitative data using a pen profile assessment and examined where the research study may have impacted the subjects.

Data Analysis

There were two methods for data analysis that were used for this research study. Quantitative analysis will be in the form of scores on the *CSQ-R* (Appendix A). Pre and post results were compared using paired t-tests, a method comparing the means of the scores before and after the yoga and art therapy interventions. The Cronbach's Alpha test was also implemented in order to determine the reliability of the assessment. Qualitative analysis was gathered from theme recognition taken from reflective journal entries regarding the yoga and the process of art making.

Risks

There were minimal risks associated with this study. However, the potential risks for this study included: feeling uncomfortable using the art materials, discomfort exposing personal information in regard to the artwork, and physical injury during the yoga practice. Additional risks included potential emotional distress as the result of the subjects being explored in the art-making process, as well as fear or frustration in regard to their own creative abilities.

The purpose of the yoga and art intervention in this study was to gauge if there was an impact on creativity and well-being. Adverse emotional reactions were not anticipated or reported post study. The participants were protected from risks during the yoga practice by the guidance of a trained yoga teacher. There was a final *Debriefing Statement* (Appendix H) that included information for local therapists and counselors. In accordance with the guidelines set forth by AATA, APA, and Notre Dame de Namur to protect the research participants, all participants signed an *Informed Consent Forms* (Appendix G), noting the voluntary nature of their participation.

Benefits

There were many potential benefits experienced by participating in this research study, including: creative flow, improved well-being, increased mind-body awareness and stress reduction. Most importantly, the participants had the opportunity to gain new skills that included increased focus and self-acceptance. Participants were also provided the opportunity to learn how to use yoga and mediation as a method for promoting health and relaxation. Additional benefits included developing a comfort level with a therapeutic practice while working within a group dynamic. There was no monetary compensation for participation in this research study.

Confidentiality

Due to the voluntary nature of study the subjects were allowed to leave the study at any time. The subjects' identities were kept anonymous throughout the entire data collection and analysis process. The records from this study will remain confidential and no individuals will be identified in any reports or publications resulting from the study. All questionnaires, artwork and journals are coded with a number that matches the corresponding consent forms and manila envelopes. All forms and number keys are stored separately from all questionnaires, test and artwork. Materials are accessible to the principal investigator and researcher supervisor only and stored in a secured file. All research information is kept by the researcher for three years and used only for research purposes. Unless published, all artwork and testing information will be destroyed after the three-year period.

Debriefing and Protection of Human Participants

At the end of the three sessions, a *Debriefing Statement* (Appendix H) was distributed to the participants with the researcher's contact information, as well as referral information for additional mental health care services if needed. The research study followed the ethical guidelines of Notre Dame de Namur University, the American Association for Marriage and Family Therapy (AAMFT), and the Art Therapy Credentials Board (ATCB). The research proposal was submitted and approved by the Institutional Review Board for approval before the research was conducted.

Implications

Based on theoretical research, this study offers the potential of providing insight into the benefits and effects of yoga and art therapy, and their prospective relationship to the creative process. It has the potential for strengthening the creative process as well as the mind-body connection, and improves participants' overall sense of well-being.

Chapter IV

Results

In this chapter, the results of the study are presented using a variety of methods. The student researcher examined the outcomes of the investigation through the lens of descriptive data, quantitative data and qualitative data.

Re-Statement of Hypotheses

The present study explored yoga's effect on the creative process. More specifically, the researcher gained valuable information regarding the specific changes in the creativity styles of adults after an intervention of Hatha Yoga. The primary investigator hypothesized that integrating the principles of positive psychology and mindfulness, alongside a practice of Hatha Yoga would have an impact on creativity. The secondary hypotheses was that the act of practicing yoga and meditation, combined with the art directives would be beneficial to strengthening the mind-body connection and improving overall well-being in participants, as well as aid in stress reduction.

Descriptive data is presented first in an effort to depict the study's participants. Following descriptive statistics is the qualitative data. The qualitative data was studied by means pen profiling and journal responses were divided into two categories: cognitive related themes and physiology related themes. This analysis will explore the significance and correlations of the assessment used in the study.

Descriptive Data

Analysis of the demographic survey provided a clear understanding of the active population. A result of eighteen volunteer participants completed the three-week yoga course. The survey collected multiple facets of descriptive data including age, gender, race/ethnicity, education, marital and employment status. Participants were able to self-report their own race/ethnicity or choose from multiple pre-selected races or ethnicities provided by this student researcher. The age range of the participants varied from 18 years old to 64 years old and the median age of the sample was 35.1. The population age was divided into five subgroups; 27.8% (n = 5) were between the ages of 18-24 years, 27.8% (n = 5) were between the ages of 25-34, 16.7% (n = 3) were between the ages of 35-44, 22.2% (n = 4) were between the ages of 45-54, and 5.5% (n = 1) were between the ages of 55-64 (Figure 1). Thirteen of the participants were female (72.2%) and five were male (27.8%) (Figure 2).

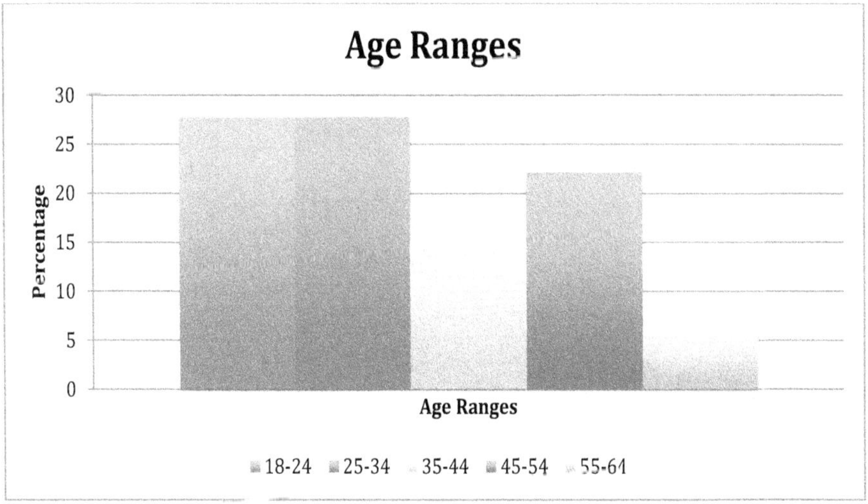

Figure 1. Graph Outlining the Range of Ages Among Participants (n = 18).

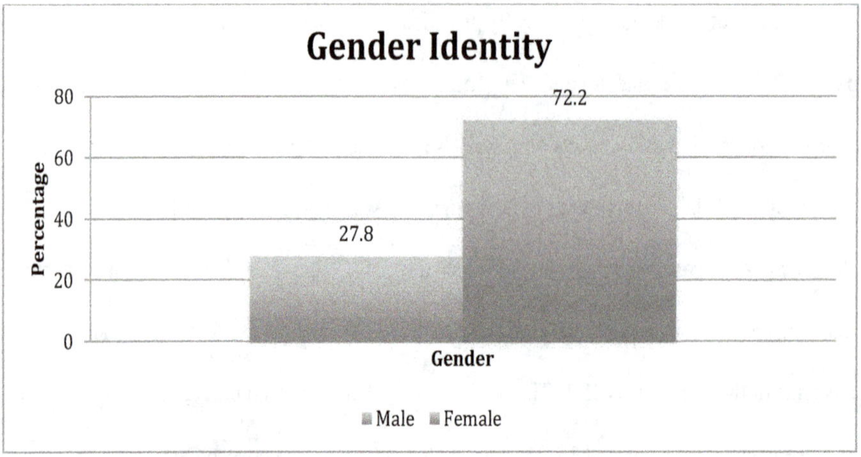

Figure 2. Graph Portraying Gender Identity of Participants (n = 18).

For this study, the participant's ethnic or racial background was also collected. The population sample consisted of a range of ethnicities. 72.2% (n = 13) identified as White/Caucasian, 11.1% (n = 2) identified as Asian/Pacific Islander, 11.1% (n = 2) identified as Latino/Latina and 5.6% (n = 1) identified as Black/African American (Figure 3).

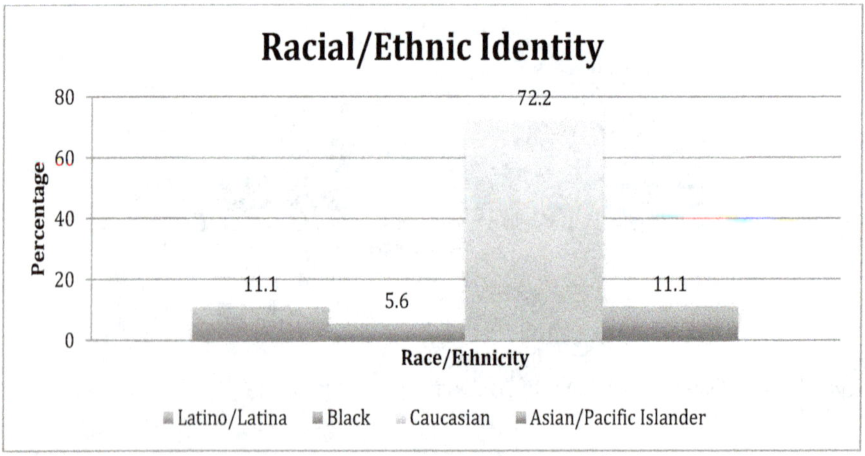

Figure 3. Graph Outlining Participants' Ethnic Identity (n = 18).

Additionally participants were asked to report on their marital status and level of education. 44.4% (n = 8) reported being married, 44.4% (n = 8) reported being single, 5.6% (n = 1) identified as being single or divorced and 5.6% (n = 1) stated that none of the categories were applicable (NA) (Figure 4). The data also reported a large range of levels of education and occupations among participants. 27.8% had Bachelor's Degrees (n = 5), 16.6 % reported vocational training, 11.1% had received a Master's Degree (n = 2), 11.1% reported having an Associate's Degree (n=2), 11.1% received some college (n = 2), 11.1% received some college but did not acquire a degree (n=2), and the remaining 10% (n = 1) had some college education, 5.6% (n=1) identified as having a professional degree and 5.6% (n = 1) reported having a Ph.D. (Figure 5).

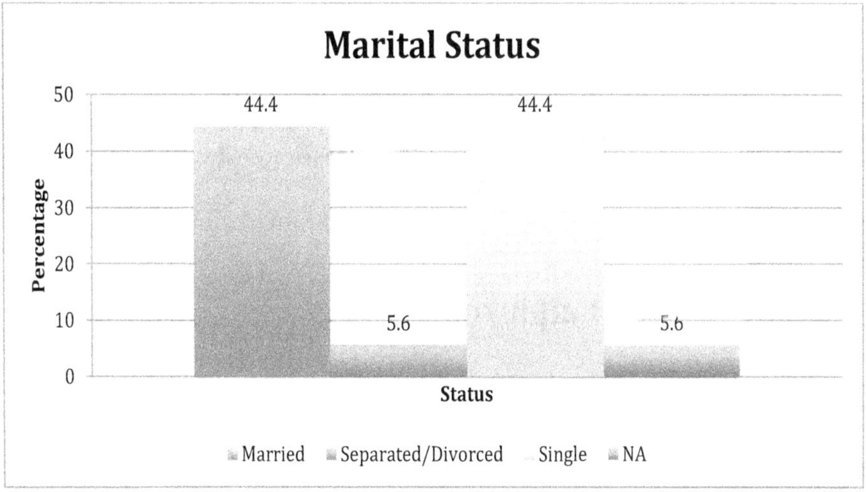

Figure 4. Graph Portraying the Marital Status of Participants (n = 18).

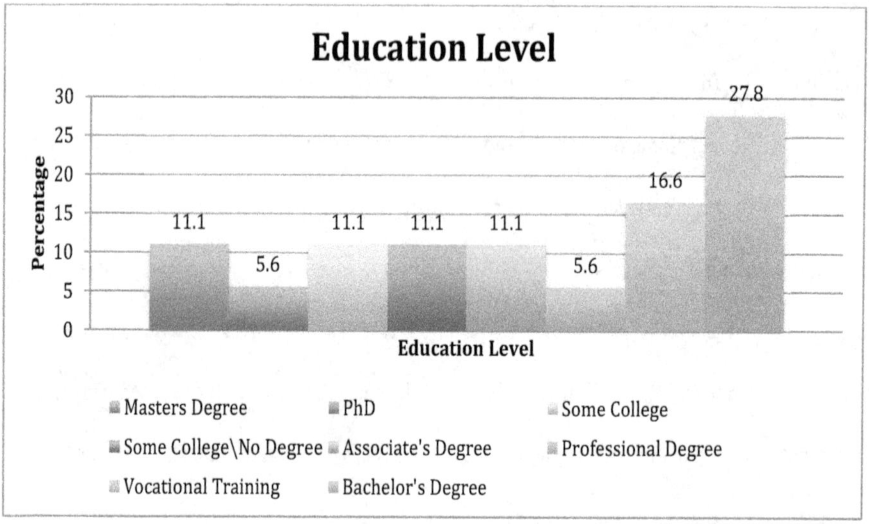

Figure 5. Graph Outlining Participants' Level of Education (n=18).

Finally, the researcher asked participants to state their employment status. There was a range of experience but 44.4% of participants (n = 8) were employed for wages while 33.3% (n = 6) identified as students, 16.7% (n = 3) reported being self-employed and 5.6% were retired (Figure 6).

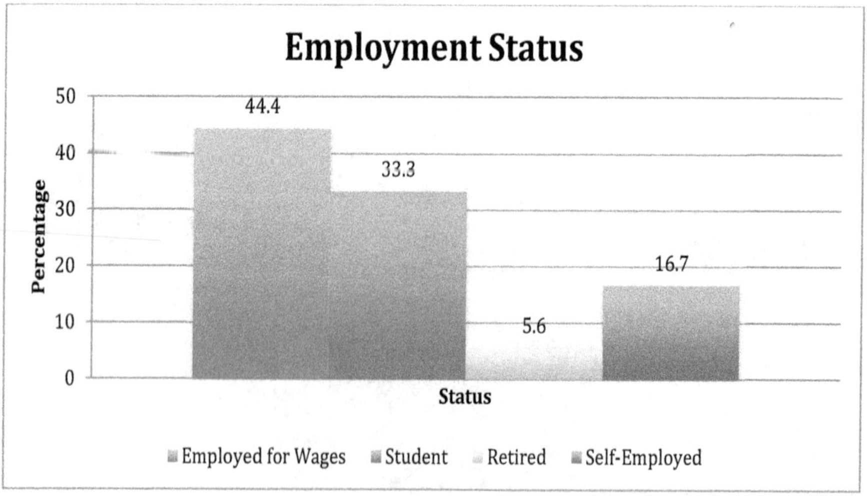

Figure 6. Graph Portraying Participants' Employment Statuses (n = 18).

Quantitative Analysis

Quantitative data was collated using the *CSQ-R* (Appendix A). The questionnaire consists of seventy-eight questions that reflect the eights scales and utilizes a likert scale answering system with Strongly Agree (1), Agree (2), Unsure (3), Disagree (4), and Strongly Disagree (5) (Kumar, Kemmler & Holman, 1997). First the pre-post test deltas were compared for each subscale between the nine participants in both the experimental group and the control group. When using a paired sample t-test to compare the pre-post test delta scores of the CSQ-R, there was significant change found in subscales T5, T7 and T8. In the experimental groups, T5 fell significantly from pre to post (Figure 7). T7 rose significantly from pre to post (Figure 9), and T8 rose significantly from pre to post (Figure 10). There were no significant changes in the control group on any of the scales.

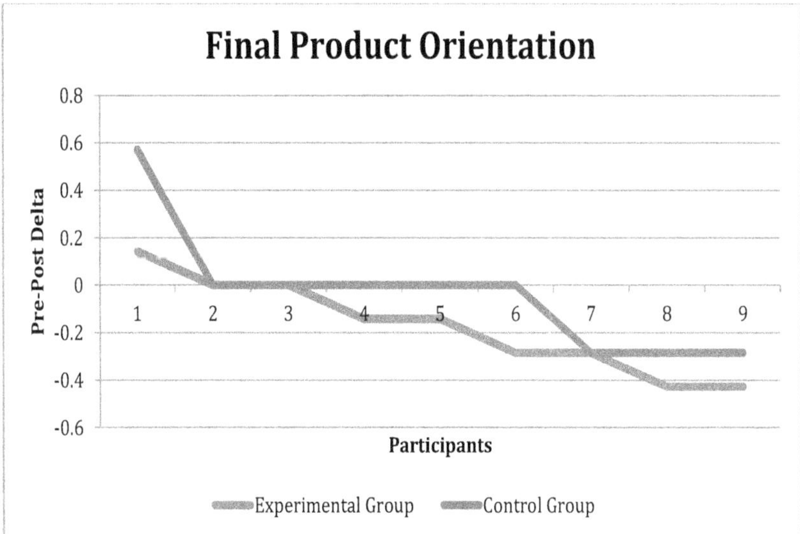

Figure 7. Graph Comparing Pre-Post Test Deltas in T5 (Final Product Orientation).

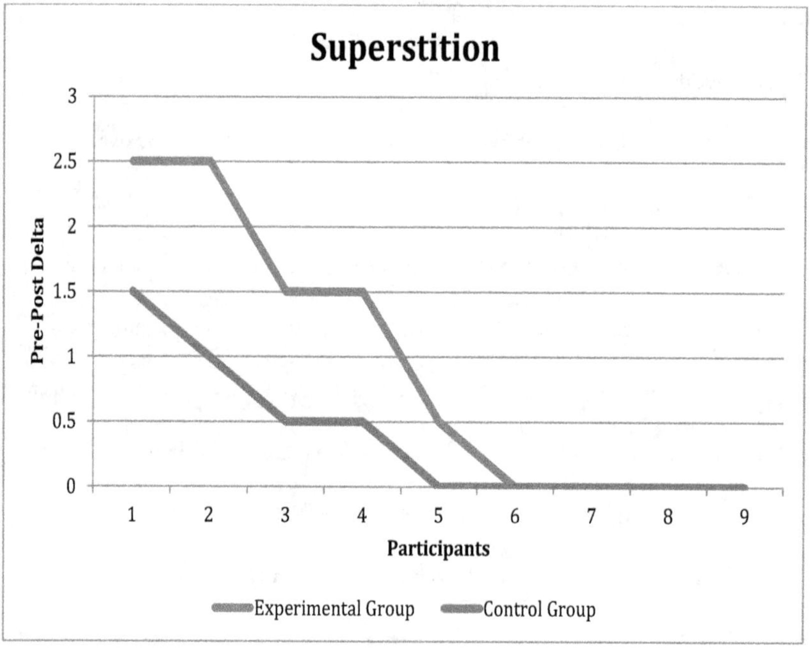

Figure 8. Graph Comparing Pre-Post Test Deltas in T7 (Superstition).

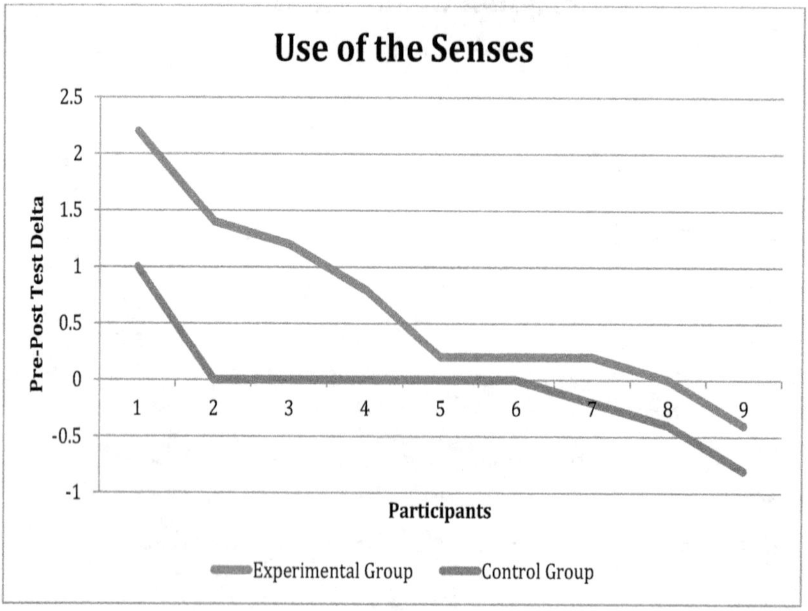

Figure 9. Graph Comparing Pre-Post Test Deltas in T8 (Use of the Senses).

Next, a paired t-test/parametric test was chosen a method for data analysis in order to compare the each of the eight mean scores on the subscale from both the experimental group and the control group. The significance threshold for this study was set at .05. Eight tests were run for each subscale to represent the changes found over the eight scales; because the CSQ-R does not provide an overall score, each of these were run separately. The table below reflects each scale within the assessment and its associated test code (Table 1).

Table 1. CSQ-R Scale Guide

Scale	Test Code
Kumar & Holman's Global Measure of Creative Capacity	T1
Belief in Unconscious Process	T2
Use of Techniques	T3
Use of Other People	T4
Final Product Orientation	T5
Environmental Control/Behavioral Self-Regulation	T6
Superstition	T7
Use of the Senses	T8

Significant differences were found among the experimental group in T5 ($p<.030$), T7 ($p<.030$), and T8 ($p<.047$), but not in the control group. Aside from these three variables, no significant changes were observed in either the experimental group or the control group; however there were a few odd results. T3 and T6 rose from pre to post for the experiment group but fell from pre to post for the control group, although neither change was found to be statistically significant. This was an unexpected result, but not of considerable importance considering that neither the experimental nor control group means of these two variables were found to be statistically significant. For the other three variables with insignificant differences, T1, T2, T4, the direction of the pre-to-post change was the same for both the experimental and control group. T1 and T2 rose from pre to post for both the experimental and control groups, and

T4 fell from pre to post for both the experimental and control groups; however none of these rises or falls were found to be statistically significant.

Table 2. Paired T-Test for Experimental and Control Group

	Experimental Group (pre & post)		Control Group (pre & post)	
Tests (# of items)	Mean of difference (pre-post)	p-value	Mean of difference (pre-post)	p-value
T1 (2 items: Q1-Q2)	-.667	.195	-.111	.594
T2 (17 items: Q3-Q19)	-.667	.723	-.556	.684
T3 (18 items: Q20-Q37)	-4.111	.312	.556	.325
T4 (9 items: Q38-Q46)	1.333	.535	.778	.244
T5 (7 items: Q47-Q53)	1.222	.030	.222	.729
T6 (18 items: Q54-Q71)	-2.444	.244	.444	.377
T7 (2 items: Q72-Q73)	-1.889	.030	-.778	.065
T8 (5 items: Q74-Q78)	-3.222	.047	.222	.787

Qualitative Results: Pen Profiles

The qualitative data (journal entries) from the participants in the experimental group underwent an initial deductive content analysis utilizing pre-identified themes from the mindfulness and flow literature to organize quotes and generate a frequency count of common themes (Patton, 2002). An inductive data analysis then took place to identify any new emergent themes. The qualitative survey was represented in the form of pen profiles and participants' verbatim quotes. Pen profiles provided a diagram of composite key emergent themes from the content analysis, frequency data, and corresponding examples from the verbatim transcripts. Within the discussion section further illustrations are offered through the use of verbatim quotes.

Cognitive Related Themes

A number of cognitive related themes were identified from participants' in the experimental group (Figure 10). Participants reported increases in relaxation (n = 15) in general throughout the yoga program: "I'm finding myself having an easier time relaxing and concentrating on myself and my body. I'm making better choices throughout the day." (Participant 5). Participants also perceived a strengthening of mind-body awareness (n = 13): "I am feeling more in tune with my body and less stressed. I find myself looking forward to these meetings every week." (Participant 6). It was also reported that some participants felt more overall acceptance for themselves (Participant 8) and appreciation for their bodies (Participant 1).

Increases in well-being and stress reduction following the yoga practice were another two common cognitive related themes. Well-being (n = 12) included a greater sense of happiness and gratitude: "When I leave the program I feel like I'm floating. I feel so happy and grateful-gratitude for myself and for those around me." (Participant 6). Stress reduction (n = 12) consequently helped some participant achieve feelings and sensations of stability, positivity and calmness: "I believe the practice is helping me reduce stress. I feel calmer when I leave and those positive feelings last throughout the rest of the day and sometimes longer." (Participant 2).

There were perceived enhancements to creative ideation (n = 7), with participant reports of feeling "highly creative" (Participant 9) and "more expressive" (Participant 6). One participant stated “Throughout these weeks I've felt less burdened by the day to day tasks. When we finish the yoga and go into the art I feel energized and inspired. I'm in the zone.” (Participant 2). In addition there were perceived improvements in the ability to concentrate (n = 6) both in the program and outside: “I am someone who is easily distracted and this program really helped me improve concentration. I was able to focus for longer and really sit with my thoughts and emotions.” (Participant 7).

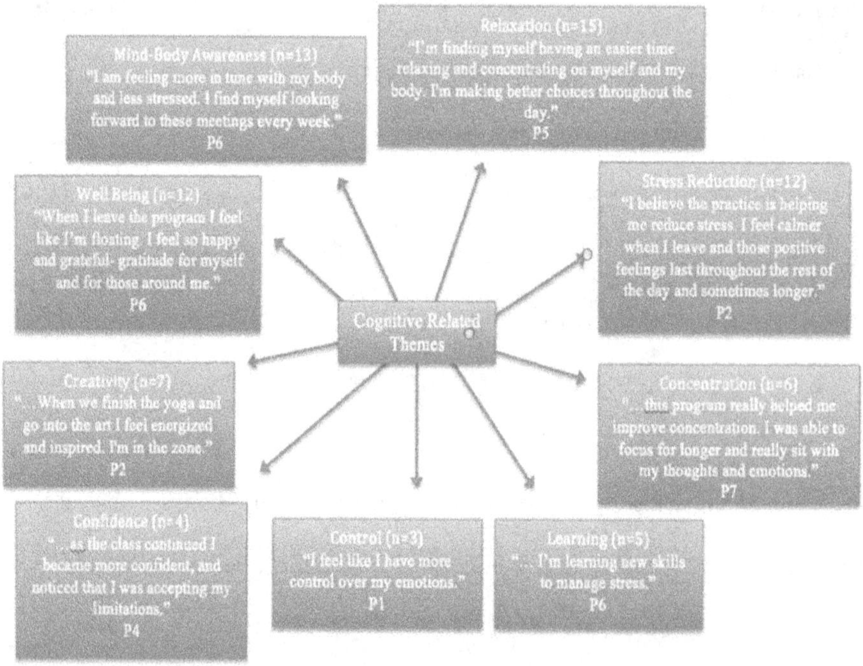

Figure 10. Cognitive-related themes identified from participants’ data with supporting examples from verbatim quotes.

Improvements in learning (n = 5) and confidence (n = 4) were also perceived, facilitating greater self-assurance and understanding. One participant reported that they were “… learning new skills to manage stress” (Participant 6). Another stated: “…as the class continued I became more confident, and noticed that I was accepting my limitations." (Participant 4). Lastly there were perceived improvements in control (n = 3). Participants reported being able to control their thoughts and feelings: "I feel like I have more control over my emotions." (Participant 1).

Physiology Related Themes

A series of physiology related themes were identified in the journal entries from the participants in the experimental group (Figure 11). Of these, feeling an increase in relaxation (n = 10) was most frequently cited, supporting previous research showing a yoga practice to elicit the relaxation response: "The yoga allowed me to feel more relaxation in my muscles." (Participant 4).

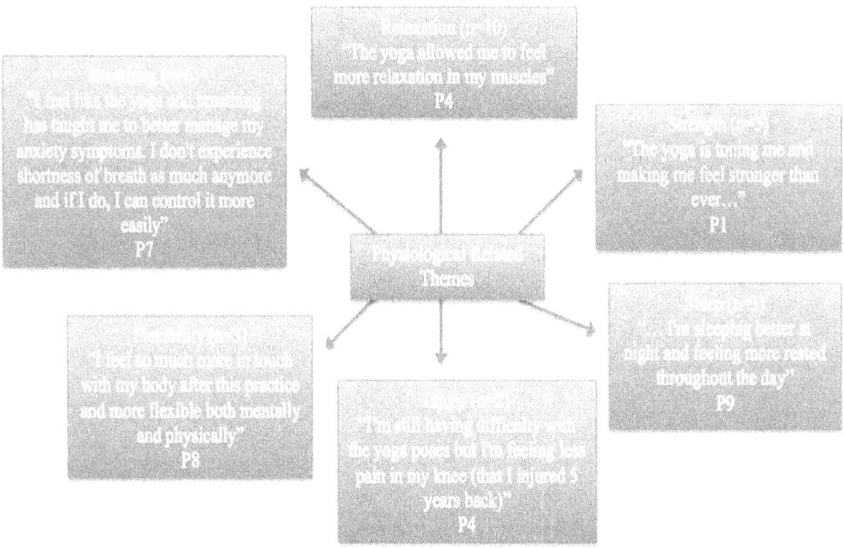

Figure 11. Physiology-related themes identified from participants' data with supporting examples from verbatim quotes.

Participants also reported improvements in breathing (n = 6) with regard to being able to control their breath more efficiently. It was suggested by one participant that these breathing improvements positively impacted her feelings of anxiety: "I feel like the yoga and breathing has taught me to better manage my anxiety symptoms. I don't experience shortness of breath as much anymore and if I do, I can control it more easily." (Participant 7).

An improvement in strength (n = 5) was another report made by participants: "The yoga is toning me and making me feel stronger than ever…" (Participant 1). Participants also revealed improvements in their quality of sleep (n = 3) and flexibility (n = 3). One participant stated "… I'm sleeping better at night and feeling more rested throughout the day." (Participant 9). Another remarked "I feel so much more in touch with my body after this practice and more flexible both mentally and physically." (Participant 8). Finally, yoga also had an impact on injury (n = 2) with participants perceiving improvements in past injurious areas of the body. One participant wrote "I'm still having difficulty with the yoga poses but I'm feeling less pain in my knee (that I injured 5 years back)." (Participant 4).

Summary

These results support both the primary and secondary hypotheses that (1) The intervention would have an impact on creativity (2) The intervention would be beneficial to strengthening the mind-body connection and improving overall well-being in participants, as well as aid in stress reduction.

Chapter V

Discussion

In the present study, the student researcher examined whether or not a three-week yoga and meditation practice would have an impact on the creative process. Eighteen adults were asked to complete multiple measures including the CSQ-R, a demographic survey and a series of journal questions created by the student researcher to measure the effectiveness of the yoga treatment. This chapter will expand upon the results as reported in the previous chapter. Additionally, the results in context of the hypotheses, future implications, and limitations will be discussed.

Re-Statement of Hypotheses

The hypotheses are (1) The integration of positive psychology, mindfulness and Hatha Yoga will have an impact on creativity (2) Practicing yoga and meditation will strengthen the mind-body connection, improve overall well-being and aid in stress reduction.

Data Interpretation

From the qualitative data, the most significant reports were the differences found among the experimental group in T5, T7 and T8, but not in the control group. T5 represents the scale of Final Product Orientation, or the extent to which people are motivated to engage in creative work by the development of a final product. T7 represents the scale of Superstition, and describes the extent to which a person engages in superstitious thoughts or behavior to facilitate creative work. T8 signifies the scale of Use of the Senses, or the extent to which a person uses the five senses for creative work (Kumar, Kemmler & Holman, 1997).

In the experimental group T5 fell significantly from pre to post, showing that as individuals participated in the yogic intervention, the product of art making became less valued than the process of creation. A possible explanation for this could be the autotelic characteristics of flow and its relationship to intrinsic motivation. As mentioned previously, Csikszentmihalyi writes that flow is autotelic or that it is an end or purpose in itself (Csikszentmihalyi, 1990, p. 67). If flow is driven and sustained by an internal reward system then this could describe why the yoga practitioners felt less compelled by the final the product over the course of the intervention.

T7 was another area that saw significant change from pre to post test. The increase in superstition indicates that participants saw an increase in superstitious thoughts or behavior to facilitate creative work. There are many different definitions of superstition, one of which is: "An excessively credulous belief in and reverence for the supernatural." (Superstition, Definition of superstition in English by Oxford Dictionaries). Mystical or transcendent experiences are widely interpreted as evidence of spirituality and have been sought throughout history through practices such as yogic meditation. Traditional yoga writings have similarly proposed that supernatural abilities have been associated with the development of spirituality (Chaube, 2015). The fact that Hatha Yoga and meditation are both components of spiritual practices that turn the mind inward, could be a possible explanation for why the yoga practitioners saw an increase in superstition.

T8 saw the most dramatic rise from pre to post, indicating a greater use of the sense in the yogic group. This factor could be the result of many things. As mentioned before, much of the literature on the benefits of yoga suggests that it increases self-awareness in practitioners (Ivtzan & Papantoniou, 2014). More specifically, the combination of mindful breathing, intentional movements and deliberate relaxation can result in sensory integration. Perhaps it is this underlying integration process that encourages mastery of the senses, and the employment of sensory engagement for creative work. This could describe the significant changes found from the pre to post test scores in the experimental group.

The qualitative data displayed similar correlations to the quantitative evidence. Following the intervention, participants reported increases in relaxation, mind-body awareness, overall well-being and less perceived stress than before the intervention. Participants also reported improvements in breath control and physical strength. The yogic group exhibited increases in use of the senses and showed a tendency toward greater control ability compared to the control group.

This study adds to the growing body of support for positive psychological approaches that emphasize the importance of happiness and human flourishing. The researcher hypothesized that the practice of yoga would have an impact on the creative process, and this study provides evidence in support of that hypothesis. The results of this study provide preliminary support for yoga as a tool for initiating flow states.

Theoretical Relationship

Positive psychology is influenced by humanistic psychology and was designed with the intention of building a more complete picture of human experience. Positive psychology is primarily concerned with individual strengths, and determining what contributes to well-being and the alleviation of human suffering (Froh, 2004). Flow, being a key function of positive psychology, is referred to as a state of optimal attention and engagement (Csikszentmihalyi, Nakamura, 2001). Flow is a dynamic state that is linked to both creativity and well-being, and is therefor a vital element to the field of art therapy. Art therapists facilitate healing and personal growth by helping individuals enter and maintain flow states. Some of the goals of art therapy are to create and identify personal meaning, promote engagement, mastery and flow, and to increase resilience and positive emotions (Arrington, 2001).

As previously discussed in the literature review, fostering creativity and increasing well-being are primary goals in both positive psychology and art therapy. In addition to these similarities, flow and art therapy also emphasize mastery as a tool for building resilience and self-esteem. The findings of this study reflect the benefits of using positive psychology and art therapy with adults. Used in conjunction, positive psychology and art therapy have the potential to become an effective vehicle for exploring the complexity of positive human experiences.

Reliability and Validity

The internal reliability of the seventy-eight item scale was examined using Cronbach's Alpha. Cronbach's Alpha ranges from 0 to 1, with higher values indicating greater internal reliability (and ultimately consistency). The alpha coefficients for the eight subscales are listed below (Table 2). None of the Cronbach's alphas were in an acceptable range (Note that a reliability coefficient of .70 or higher is considered acceptable in most social science research situations). Although the results indicate that the CSQ-R has relatively low internal consistency, these indices in the CSQ-R have been studied and applied extensively in psychometrics literature. Low internal reliability occurs for various reasons.

In this study, I believe the main factor that negatively impacted the internal consistency was due to the small number of observations. Although the results of this investigation are generally positive, it suffers from flaws that are relatively common for research in real working environments. Additionally, the CSQ-R is considered an industry standard in the field of creativity research. The psychometrics research is extensive and verifies that the questionnaire has high validity and is overall a trusted assessment.

Table 3. Cronbach's Alpha Reliability Pre-Test Report

Scale	Cronbach's Alpha	N of Items
T1: Kumar & Holman's Global Measure of Creative Capacity (Q1-Q2)	0.572	2
T2: Belief in Unconscious Process (Q3-19)	0.429	17
T3: Use of Techniques (Q20-Q37)	0.523	18
T4: Use of Other People (Q38-46)	0.632	9
T5: Final Product Orientation (Q47-Q53)	-0.080	7
T6: Environmental Control/Behavioral Self-Regulation (Q54-Q71)	0.873	18
T7: Superstition (Q72-73)	0.444	2
T8: Use of the Senses (Q74-Q78)	0.434	5

Table 4. Cronbach's Alpha Reliability Post-Test Report

Scale	Cronbach's Alpha	N of Items
T1: Kumar & Holman's Global Measure of Creative Capacity (Q1-Q2)	.146	2
T2: Belief in Unconscious Process (Q3-19)	.367	17
T3: Use of Techniques (Q20-Q37)	.473	18
T4: Use of Other People (Q38-46)	.566	9
T5: Final Product Orientation (Q47-Q53)	-.011	7
T6: Environmental Control/Behavioral Self-Regulation (Q54-Q71)	.852	18
T7: Superstition (Q72-73)	.661	2
T8: Use of the Senses (Q74-Q78)	.397	5

Limitations and Recommendations for Future Research

The findings of this study should be interpreted in light of several limitations that preclude definitive conclusions. There are three primary limitations of the study that are to be noted while interpreting the results. First, the reliability of the instrument was low. It is not clear as to why the reliability of this scale was low, even though many results were in the expected direction. The researcher theorizes that low reliability may have occurred for two reasons. The first is due to the small sample size and the second is that the participants were asked to respond to a large number of questions in a relatively small time frame. Studying a small population reduced the power of the study and increased the margin of error. This is perhaps the greatest limitation for it potentially undermined the reliability of the study and skewed the results. Collecting a larger sample size was the desired goal, but ultimately the study was limited due to time constraints, scheduling conflicts and fiscal impediments. Some solutions to this problem would be a longer time frame for the study and financial resources to fund the research. Future researchers can avoid this problem by expanding the sample size and by allotting more time for respondents to complete the creativity instrument.

Second, the generalizability of the study is limited by the use of convenience sampling. Implementing this method provided the researcher with participants from a specific group of people but does not provide data that is representative of the larger population. Hence, some groups were over-represented and some were under-represented. This in turn creates biased data, making the study more prone to inaccuracies and sampling errors. Ultimately using this method made it impossible to acquire generalized conclusions and using alternative means of sampling is encouraged in future research.

Finally the overall lack of diversity found in the population, particularly in regard to gender and ethnicity. The sample had a disproportionate number of females compared to males. Similarly, there was a large percent of the population that identified as white or Caucasian. The researcher believes that these results reflect the larger trend in the United States. According to 2016 Yoga in America study, eighty-two percent of yoga practitioners identified as female and eighteen percent identified as male (Yoga Journal, 2016). For this reason, finding methods of appealing to males and people of ethnically diverse backgrounds would be crucial to generating generalizable data. Perhaps advertising differently in future studies would ensure the appeal to both sexes and would allow for more variation of data.

Union of Yoga and Art Therapy in Clinical Practice

The practice of yoga corresponds in several ways to the field of art therapy. A growing body of research supports the claim that yoga can improve physiological functioning as well as psychological functioning including: reductions in stress, anxiety and depression and improve relaxation, focus, and self-esteem (Ross & Thomas, 2010). Similarly, art therapy has been shown to be rehabilitative and transformational. Art making engages both the motor and sensory pathways of one's neurology. Evidence shows how art making with intention, and professionally-informed therapeutic direction engages both the left and right hemispheres of the brain, as well as the cerebellum (Wilkinson & Chilton, 2013). This type of art making allows individuals to process difficult emotions and feelings that can then lead to greater understanding and healing. The individual who is engaged in the art making process is thinking, feeling, processing and responding to the entire experience of art therapy.

Combining the two healing modalities of yoga and art therapy in clinical practice creates a non-invasive, holistic, multi-sensory healing experience that both activates and protects the individual throughout the healing journey. The yoga, breath work and meditation help to relax and open the physical body, while the art making provides access to a less guarded, less self-conscious part of the self. It is this researcher's view that implementing the use of art therapy in this state makes self-expression and self-reflection more likely to occur. Embracing yoga as a complement to art therapy could enhance the field's efficacy, and encourage individuals and clinicians to implement yoga as a coping tool to be used both inside and outside the therapeutic environment.

Conclusion

Despite the limitations, the findings of this study indicate that yoga and meditation had a significant impact on creativity. The results specify four primary components that were altered by the yogic intervention. According to the present study, engagement in the yoga program altered the perceived importance of the final product (mandala art intervention), moving away from extrinsic motivation and toward intrinsic motivation. It also increased participants perceived belief that superstitious thoughts and behaviors are needed to facilitate creative work. Additionally, the most dramatic change from the qualitative data indicated a greater use of the sense in the yogic group. Finally, the examination of participants' pen profiles indicated signs of stress reduction and increases in relaxation, mind-body awareness and well-being.

The results of this study are consistent with previous research and offers insight into the use of yoga for initiating flow and increasing mind-body awareness in adults. Furthermore, these results could benefit art therapists who seek to explore the unique benefits of the art therapy process to generate mastery of flow, to improve mood, and to create meaning in life. This study supports the claim that art therapy should be used as a method to encourage creative flow and overall well-being. More studies are needed and future researchers should consider using a randomized, longitudinal study around the conjoined use of yoga and art therapy approaches in research and practice. This approach would work to demonstrate specific outcomes and to gain a better understanding of the complex interplay between the mind-body connection and art therapy. In the final analysis of the results of this study, the investigator provided preliminary support for the efficacy of a brief yogic intervention that incorporates mindfulness techniques alongside art directives. The researcher highlighted the potential benefits and defended the reasons why the subject deserves to have continued exploration within this novice field of promising treatment.

Statement of Personal Interest

My interest in flow began at an early age and became more developed from my yoga and art practices. The compatibility between yoga and art was always clear, but it wasn't until I began studying art therapy that the expansive potential for healing was uncovered. As a researcher I am primarily interested in exploring the cognitive neuroscience of creativity and human flourishing. In the future I hope to better understand the underlying neurocognitive correlates of flow in the context of the field. Based on the research I've completed thus far I have confidence that art therapy and yoga-based practices (YBP) are fundamentally working toward the same goals: self-awareness, self-regulation, and self-acceptance.

As a mental health professional in a young field, I'm optimistic in using yoga and art therapy in conjunction to open up new possibilities for practice. I believe that teaching individuals how to utilize flow to find authentic happiness could bring about several benefits including: the establishment of holistic, preventative measures for mental illness, the reduction of stigmas around mental health, and the increase in curiosity about the mind-body connection. This master's thesis is the first step in my exploration of the relationship between yoga, flow and art therapy.

CPSIA information can be obtained
at www.ICGtesting.com
Printed in the USA
LVHW021641120423
744200LV00009B/303

9 788097 135454